MW01027665

NATURE'S IMMUNE ENHANCER

Echinacea, the most popular and effective remedy in the herbal medicine chest, is enjoying a renaissance in the United States today, lining the shelves not only of natural food stores, but more conventional pharmacies as well.

Yet, echinacea once enjoyed an even greater popularity in America. In this fascinating book, a distinguished herbalist tells the little-known story of echinacea, tracing its popularity in the late 19th century, its subsequent fall from grace and its eventual rebirth 100 years later: a story which illustrates one of the most intriguing chapters in American medical history.

Drawing on years of research and study, Dr. Mowrey also discusses the many uses of echinacea not only as an immune stimulant, but as an antiviral, antifungal and antibiotic agent as well as its healing properties in disorders of the respiratory system, the skin and the inflammation of arthritis. Dr. Mowrey concludes his comprehensive report with practical information on how to grow echinacea, known to gardeners as the beautiful plant, purple coneflower, and how to make your own extract.

ABOUT THE AUTHOR

Daniel B. Mowrey, Ph.D., one of America's most respected researchers and writers in the field of herbalism, is Director of the American Phytotherapy Research Laboratory in Salt Lake City. Among his many published books are *Herbal Tonic Therapies, Proven Herbal Blends, Next Generation Herbal Medicine* and *The Scientific Validation of Herbal Medicine,* also published by Keats Publishing, Inc.

ECHINACEA

HOW AN AMAZING HERB SUPPORTS AND STIMULATES YOUR IMMUNE SYSTEM

by Daniel B. Mowrey, Ph.D.

Keats Publishing, Inc. New Canaan, Connecticut

Echinacea is not intended as medical advice. Its intent is solely informational and educational. Please consult a health professional should the need for one be indicated.

ECHINACEA

ISBN: 0-87983-610-5

Printed in the United States of America

Good Health Guides are published by
Keats Publishing, Inc.
27 Pine Street (Box 876)
New Canaan, Connecticut 06840-0876

CONTENTS

INTRODUCTION

A new and remarkable medicinal plant burst upon the scene in the late 1980s. It even caught the imagination of the popular press and was recommended for the common cold by many American physicians. It possessed a name difficult to pronounce and remember and it was commonly known to botanists as purple coneflower. That quaint and descriptive name, however, was not to become the popular term for the plant. Instead, manufacturers, herbalists and the public all agreed to call the plant by its botanical designation, *echinacea*, pronounced ECK-I-NAY-SE-AH. Echinacea has now become the common name for several echinacea species, including *E. angustifolia*, *E. purpurea*, and *E. pallida*. But, despite the intense curiosity and infatuation exhibited by the modern user, echinacea is not new; it once enjoyed an even greater popularity in America. How that happened, how the herb descended into obscurity and what gave rise to its current renaissance will be reviewed in this book. We will also describe current uses of the plant in treating a wide range of complaints, especially in connection with the immune system.

THE ECHINACEA STORY: A HISTORY

The story of the discovery of echinacea as a medicinal plant and its formal introduction to the medical community forms one of the more interesting chapters in American medical history. The 1800s witnessed the rise of at least four major medical movements in this country. The orthodox allopaths, or "regulars," who were caught up in the use of various "heroic" medicines such as blood letting that probably killed more people than they cured; the Thomsonians, who rebelled against the regulars by employing herbal preparations exclusively, some of which were almost as drastic as the heroic drugs; the eclectics, who employed what they considered the best cures and medicines available, no matter what the source; and the homeopaths, a group of physicians practicing homeopathy, a very dilute form of herbal medicine invented in Germany, which was an increasingly popular reaction against allopathy or regular medicine during the 1800s. All four groups used herbal medicines, but as time went on, the Thomsonians lost favor, the eclectics enjoyed perhaps the greatest degree of success, the homeopaths maintained popularity, and the regulars went about consolidating the power needed to eliminate all forms of competition.

Against this background of multiple schools of medicine, it was not uncommon for men to assume the mantle of doctor on the most flimsy of rationales. Self-taught physicians roamed the American frontier, questionable medical schools dotted the landscape, and doctors waged war with one another over the viability of ideas, cures, treatments and methods. This was the age of the "patent medicines," which were not really patented at all, but were the subject of incredible claims, and were the basis of a good deal of fraudulent behavior on the part of unscrupulous characters trying to make a fast buck. The ignorance of early settlers concerning native medicinal lore contributed to the acceptance of this pharmaceutical quackery.

Meanwhile, legitimate pharmaceuticals were available, and some of the trade secrets being sold from the back of traveling covered wagons were effective medicines gleaned from the medicinal lore of the American Indian or discovered accidentally by intelligent investigators of plant materials.

In this climate, legitimate pharmaceutical manufacturers were continually being inundated with the latest "miracle cures." Pharmacists like the Lloyd Brothers of Cincinnati,

Ohio, were therefore often faced with the possibility of making either of two potentially devastating errors. One, they could accept as legitimate some obscure cure that was in fact bogus; or two, they could reject a valid treatment. The latter of the two alternatives was obviously the less risky, and hence was often the governing principle for the routine handling of inquiries received from health practitioners of the frontier.

The person most responsible for the early popularization of this herbal treatment was John Uri Lloyd, whose colorful exploits in pharmacy and literature have become legend. His description of the frontier medical environment follows:

"In no place do we find this helplessness of man in the face of nature better depicted than in that of medicine. . . . Together we of the medical profession and pharmaceutical art are treading our way, and sorting the chaff from the grain. We turn from the aborigine to the man of science. We take from one and the other; we adopt the good, reject the bad. . . . the aborigine stands conspicuous as the friend that has done the most in helpful original experimentation for the unborn science of medicine. Surely the most in the past, possibly he is doing the most in the present. Take from medicine those substances introduced to the profession by the aborigines, and those that the profession stumbled over by chance, and 'the science' would be irretrievably crippled.

"Among the most conspicuous recent examples of the empiricist's work, stands the drug Echinacea, which heads this paper, and that has a history which might well be the subject of a romance—a history that, as I unravel it from the data at my command, and which is at the command only of him who writes this paper, calls to mind vividly the method of the empiricist, and the obligation we are under to the primary empiricist (H.C.F. Meyer, Prof. John King, the Indians)."[2]

The following remarks are from a pamphlet entitled *Echinacea*, published by Lloyd Brothers, Cincinnati, Ohio, in 1923.

"**Discovery.** In the fall of 1885 I received from Dr. H.C.F. Meyer, of Pawnee City, Nebraska, the root of a plant that he wished named. He stated that he used it in making "Meyer's Blood

Purifier," a remedy heralded in large type by his letterhead. At the same time, he sent to Professor John King a bottle of the preparation, making for it the most exaggerated claims.

"Dr. Meyer's exaggerated claims in behalf of Echinacea strongly prejudiced me against it. Professor King, however, with a more comprehensive view of problems such as this, decided to give it a fair therapeutic investigation, and at his request I proceeded to institute a careful series of pharmaceutical experiments with Echinacea. Dr. King, indeed, soon developed a strong personal interest in the drug, the tincture of which was found to be a palliator in the treatment of Mrs. King, who at that time was afflicted with a virulent cancer ... who found this to be the only remedy that gave her any relief. Dr. King continued his investigations of Echinacea, becoming therefrom so convinced of its value that in 1887 he announced it to the medical profession, in a conservative, signed article, contributed to the *Eclectic Medical Journal*."

Comparing the attitudes of Dr. King and Dr. Lloyd, we can easily determine the general medical climate of the 1800s. On the one hand, Dr. Lloyd displayed the prevalent skepticism relative to plant medicines; on the other hand, Dr. King demonstrated an uncommon willingness to explore new methods or products that typified certain frontier physicians. Finally, the subsequent rapid acceptance of echinacea by eclectic (and eventually, orthodox) physicians demonstrates the openmindedness and spirit of adventure that characterized early American professionals.

In Dr. King's original article, he states that echinacea "certainly merits a careful investigation by our practitioners; and should it be found to contain only one-half the virtues he (Meyer) attributes to it, it will form an important addition to our materia medica." One suspects that the full set of purported virtues must have been quite spectacular. Dr. Lloyd gives a little flavor of what it must have been like in the following anecdote:

"Within a short time after the identification of Echinacea, Dr. Meyer wrote to Dr. King and myself, urging us to give the profession the benefit of his discovery. In view of our incredulity as to virtues of the drug in the direction of bites of poisonous serpents, he offered to come to Cincinnati and, in the presence of a committee selected by ourselves, allow a rattlesnake of our selection to bite him wherever we might prefer the wound to be inflicted, proposing then to antidote the poison by means of Echinacea only. This offer (or rather, challenge) we declined. Dr. Meyer, thinking this was because we had no serpent at our command, again offered not only to come to Cincinnati and submit to the ordeal formerly proposed, but to bring with him a full-sized rattlesnake, possessed of its natural fangs, allow it bite him repeatedly, under the auspices of a selected committee, and having them use the antidote, to demonstrate to the profession the value of Echinacea as a remedy for a human being thus inoculated. This offer was also declined."

By this we see that Dr. Meyer virtually embodied the American pioneer spirit.

Many years after the events described above, Dr. Lloyd was still chagrined at having failed to recognize the value of echinacea as quickly as did others, including Dr. King. Concerning this matter and the subsequent popularity of echinacea, Lloyd penned the following:

"Echinacea stands conspicuous in that, in the face of its exceedingly lukewarm reception by those under those auspices it was destined to be introduced, as well as pronounced resistance it met elsewhere, it has earned for itself, in the phenomenally short period of thirty years, the exceptional place it now occupies with American practicing physicians. It is today [1923] the most used American drug introduced since 1885. My own delay in its general introduction is to me now a subject of self-criticism. I am now more pronouncedly of the opinion, as experiences multiply, that a person who is restricted to laboratory experiments, especially if he be more or less adversely prejudiced (as I was against Echinacea), is not in a position to judge with discretion."

What was the extent of echinacea's reputation in these early years? Perhaps the following quote from Harvey Felter, an early eclectic physician will suffice to illustrate the fact that reports of echinacea's effectiveness were so glowing and uniformly positive that physicians were hesitant to truthfully report these data, but rather chose to downplay the plant to some degree.

"Conspicuous among the remedies introduced within recent years, echinacea undoubtedly takes the first rank. . . . As with all new remedies, it has suffered the usual over-estimation, in that it has been endorsed for almost the whole range of human ailments, and the exaggerated claims made for it led Professor Lloyd, for a long time, to view it with suspicion. Many over-sanguine statements concerning its wonderful—yes, practically impossible—virtues have, however, been judiciously withheld from publication, lest a remedy of great value should be placed in bad repute through exaggerated reports—a condition that has not been altogether avoided even by this care. But is this not the record of the majority of the most important of our drugs?"[3]

An example of the kind of writing about echinacea to which Felter refers in the above paragraph is the following, taken from *The Eclectic Medical Journal* of March, 1897. A certain J.C. Paxon, M.D., from Jamesville, Illinois, wrote as follows:

Echinacea. Mrs. P., aged 85, during winters for the past five years, has had a peculiar trouble. It begins by itching on the hands and feet so intense that it is almost unbearable, as reported to me one year ago. In spite of all treatment her physician gave, the termination was by great watery blisters, breaking down in suppurating sores. In January, 1896 . . . I placed her on echinacea . . . every hour, and to her surprise the itching began to subside by the time she had taken three doses, and she was completely relieved in 48 hours without any blisters or sores following, as had been the case the three winters previous."

On the frontier the advent of a treatment that really worked was greeted with great acclaim and was accorded the highest reputation. In the case of echinacea, however, apparently extraordinary efforts were employed to keep reports of astounding cures from the public. In just over one decade, the Eclectic Medical College in Cincinnati had collected hundreds of such reports.

It seems that whenever a new and effective medical treatment is introduced, there follows a period during which the product seemingly cures everything. Then comes a period in which careful research and observation sorts out the bogus from the authentic. Finally, given sufficient time and research interest, a unified and reliable constellation of properties is established, and the product takes its place among the standard pharmaceuticals of the medical establishment. Unfortunately, as we shall see, this process was cut short in the case of echinacea and just as the herb was about to assume a place next to quinine and other legitimate plant drugs, certain political events ended the medical use of the preparation.

Although the eclectics tried to suppress publication of clinical trials, word of this remarkable new remedy spread like wildfire. Over the next dozen years following its introduction in 1885, the popularity of echinacea continued to increase at a rapid pace. By 1898 echinacea had risen to the top of the list of popular natural treatments in America. Users included not just the eclectics, but hosts of regular doctors who recognized the virtue of herbal preparations and other holistic methods over the kind of heroic, intrusive and often deadly treatments available through orthodoxy.

An extensive review and history of echinacea, summarizing much of the early work on the plant, was written in 1898 by one of the leading proponents of eclectic medicine, H. W. Felter.[4] Excerpts from this article are presented below. Notice the wide variety of uses for which echinacea was being used at the time.

"The following range of affections were those in which Dr. Meyer claimed success for this remedy· malarial fever, *choleru morbus, cholera infantum*, boils and internal abscesses, typhoid fever (internally and locally to abdomen), ulcerated sore throat, old ulcers, poisoning from rhus, erysipelas, carbuncles, bites and stings of bees, wasps, spiders, etc., in nasal and pharyngeal catarrh, hemorrhoids, various fevers, including typhoid, congestive and remittent, trichinosis, nervous headache, acne, *scrofulous ophthalmia*, milk crust, scald head, and eczema; also colic in horses.

"Subsequent use of the drug has in a measure substantiated the seemingly incredulous claims of its introducer, for it will be observed that most of these conditions were such as might be due to blood depravation, or to noxious introductions from without the body—the very field in which echinacea is known to display its power. Goss (*Chicago Medical Times*, 1888), who also became interested in the drug, praised it as a remedy for mad-dog bites, chronic catarrh, chronic ulcers, gonorrhea, and syphilis.

"If any single statement were to be made concerning the virtues of echinacea it would read something like this: 'A corrector of the depravation of the body fluids;' and even this does not sufficiently cover the ground. Its extraordinary powers—combining essentially that formerly included under the terms antiseptic, antifermentative, and antizymotic—are well shown in its power over changes produced in the fluids of the body, whether from internal causes or from external introductions. The changes may be manifested in a disturbed balance of the fluids resulting in such tissue alterations as are exhibited in boils, carbuncles, abscesses, or cellular glandular inflammations. They may be from the introduction of serpent or insect venom, or they may be due to such fearful poisons as give rise to malignant diphtheria, cerebrospinal meningitis, or puerperal and other forms of septicaemia. 'Bad blood,' so called, asthenia and adynamia, and particularly a tendency to malignancy in acute and subacute disorders, seem to be special indicators for the use of echinacea."

"A crushed hand, thought to be beyond aid, with the intolerable stench of putrid flesh, was saved by the application of echinacea. It has given equally satisfactory results in alarming cases of venom infection, with great depression, from the bites of the rattlesnake, tarantula and other spiders, and from the stings of scorpions, bees, wasps, etc. . . . Chronic catarrhal bronchitis and fetid bronchitis have been signally benefited by echinacea, and it has done that which few remedies can accomplish, i.e., it has overcome the stench of pulmonary gangrene, and if given early it is asserted to avert a gangrenous termination in pulmonic affections."

Felter also recommended echinacea as a good appetite stimulant, to improve digestion, as a remedy for fevers and pain, as an intestinal antiseptic, as a topical dressing for malignant carbuncle and as a remedy for eczema. Much of the language of the above quotes seems strange to modern ears. Many of the infections referred to have been fairly well eradicated from the Western world, and a certain degree of evolution has occurred in the scientific and medical language employed to discuss and describe disease. Ironically, terms like alternative, blood purifier, detoxifier, antiseptic, etc., are actually more understandable and accessible to the modern reader than the complex language of physiology and immunology that is now the accepted medical parlance for actions demonstrated by echinacea.

Harvey Felter was one of the most prolific eclectics around the turn of the century. A short time after penning the above description, he wrote another treatise describing the uses, methods of application and other features of echinacea[5] (*Echinacea*, Lloyd Brothers, Pharmacists, Inc., Cincinnati, Ohio, probably somewhere between 1900–1905). Felter summarized the indications for the employment of echinacea as follows:

"Bad blood ... to correct fluid depravation, with tendency to sepsis and malignancy, best shown in its power in gangrene, carbuncles, boils, sloughing and phagedenic ulcerations, and the various forms of septicemia; ... tendency to formation of multiple cellular abscesses of a semiactive character and with pronounced asthenia; ... foul discharges with emaciation and great debility; ... dirty-brownish tongue; ... jet-black tongue; ... dusky, bluish or purplish color of the skin or mucous tissues, with a low form of inflammation."

Felter recommended echinacea in the treatment of many external and internal problems. He considered the plant to be a stimulant, deodorant and anesthetic in external diseases, and employed it as such in the treatment of conditions such as ulcerations, infections, gangrene, bed sores, wounds, foul breath, pyorrhea, aphthous and herpetic eruptions, eczema, erysipelas, chilblains and dermatitis, snake bites, insect bites and stings, urticaria, boils and carbuncles. Internally, he employed echinacea in support of all external applications. Additionally, he used the plant as a stimulant, depurative, antiseptic and antiputrefactive in the treatment of cancer, fevers of all kinds, flu, leucorrhea, indigestion and gastric pain.

"Blood depravation" was defined by Felter as "diseases which show a depraved condition of the body and its fluids." He explains further;

> "No satisfactory explanation for its action has ever been given, and that a simple drug should possess such varied and remarkable therapeutic forces and not be a poison itself is an enigma still to be solved, and one that must come as a novelty to those whose therapy is that of heroic medicines only. If there is any meaning in the term *alternative*, it is expressed in the therapy of echinacea. For this reason a most excellent medicine has been lauded extravagantly and came near to damnation through the extravagant praises of its admirers."

Felter suggested that echinacea is of great benefit

> "where the blood stream becomes slowly infected either from within or without the body. Elimination is imperfect, the body tissues become altered, and there is developed within the fluids and tissues septic action with adynamia, resulting in boils, carbuncles, cellular tissue inflammations, abscesses and other septicemic processes. It is, therefore, a drug indicated by the changes manifested in a disturbed balance of the fluids of the body, resulting in tissue alteration—be the cause infectious by organisms, or devitalized morbid accumulations, or alterations in the blood itself."

Felter qualifies this list with a few cautionary statements.

> "To assume that Echinacea will cure every type of disease because it succeeds in aiding the milder forms to recover is to bring a good medicine into unmerited discredit. Moreover, when these claims were originally made, and probably in good faith, there was no exact means of establishing the bacterial nature of the disease, hence many tonsillar disorders were called diphtheria. The latter were, of course, benefited by it, for in tonsillitis, particularly the necrotic form with stinking, dirty-looking ulcerations, it is an excellent remedy."

Felter recommends that external problems be treated with echinacea liquid extracts, some of which were iodized at the time, and with echinacea creams. Internally, liquid extracts, tinctures and combinations were recommended. The iodized preparation was specific for external use. I am unaware of a current form of echinacea containing iodine.

The life of the frontier doctor must have been exciting. Confronted on a daily basis by deadly diseases, industrial accidents, difficult pregnancies and other demanding problems, he must have been continually on the lookout for agents to relieve pain, halt epidemics, save lives, abort infections, and so forth. Into this situation came echinacea, which solely by word of mouth, not by advertising or propaganda, had already achieved an enormous reputation. Doctors must have tried it on everything. Perhaps the following exploits of a turn-of-the-century M.D., G. L. B. Rounseville, will illustrate the impact echinacea had on daily medical practice.[6] Note that the author misspells echinacea as *echinacca* throughout this paper.

"Echinacca angustifolia is a stimulant, diaphoretic, diuretic, sialagogue, cathartic and antipyretic.... Its greatest value as a restorative agent is found in the degeneration of cell tissues from microbic invasion or from septic or other poisons, where the ptomanes and leucomanes are present. That it does arrest these most dangerous septic conditions there can be no doubt.

"Rabies: I was called upon to treat two children, aged 4 and 6, who had been bitten by a rabid dog, on December 28th, 1902. Both had been bitten in the face and through the upper lip. I will not go into detail, only to say that all facts proved that the dog was rabid. I made a 50 per cent solution of Echinacca and gave 4 and 6 drop doses every four hours and followed it for nearly 60 days. The children, two girls, have evidenced no symptoms of rabies to date and I don't believe they ever will.

"I will report a case from a mechanical injury: A freight conductor whose hand had been injured several days before, while coupling cars along the line of railway of which I am surgeon.... I found the thumb, first and second fingers, together with the carpal portion of the hand, in a gangrenous condition. The bones of the three digits fractured, inflammation extending nearly to the shoulder.... After thoroughly irrigating with bichloride solution, I carefully dressed the hand with sterilized gauze, upon which I applied a roller bandage nearly to the shoulder. I made a prescription of Echinacca, and ordered one—half teaspoonful to be taken internally every two hours and to keep the bandage thoroughly saturated with the lotion. The patient returned to me the following morning, had no temperature, said he had rested well, the first sleep for three days. On taking off the dressing, the gangrenous portion sloughed out, the inflammation had subsided. I . . . gave the Echinacca for a few days internally. In one month and two days the patient reported for duty with complete recovery."

One wonders, Did the echinacea really do all of these wonderful things, or was misdiagnosis or willful deceit involved? It is hard to imagine a placebo effect so strong that it would affect the course of such serious conditions. If echinacea really worked these kinds of miracles then, could it not do so now? Such a powerful medicine should be able to easily deal with everyday infections that currently plague modern civilization.

By the end of the first decade of the twentieth century, the fame of echinacea had spread from coast to coast. Doctors, faced with a long litany of debilitating infectious diseases, discovered that echinacea would help them when other treatments failed. The Lloyd Brothers Pharmaceutical House responded to the huge demand for the substance by developing increasingly sophisticated and pure extracts.

A fascinating survey was made in 1911 by the members of house of Lloyd.[7] They asked hundreds of doctors, both eclectic and otherwise, to evaluate the relative importance of the Lloyd Bros. preparations. Echinacea was ranked fifth by eclectics, but was surprisingly ranked first by physicians other than eclectics. That echinacea would be considered more valuable by non-eclectic doctors than by members of the school claiming discovery of the medicine attests to the popularity echinacea had achieved by 1911 among American physicians in general.

From this time forward, periodic reviews of echinacea would appear in various eclectic medical journals. These reviews served as a yardstick for evaluating the evolving field of echinacea medical use. One of these reviews by Dr. J. Fearn[8] is especially valuable because it synthesized much of the early work and gave it a unified structure. Excerpts from this review are presented below.

> **"Therapy.** I believe that no remedy ever introduced into the practice of medicine, has gained such extensive use, or accomplished as much good in the same period of time as echinacea. In fevers it brings down temperatures; in fevers of an adynamic type with obstructed circulation and tendency to sepsis, it brings about normal circulation and overcomes sepsis. It acts on the three great emunctories, the skin, the kidneys and the bowels, thus opening those great flood gates for the elimination of poisonous matter, and while breaking down and eliminating poisonous matter in this way, it is a good appetizer and improves digestion, so that while tearing down it also builds up."

Fearn admits that some physicians may act too hastily in applying echinacea. This fact only serves to underscore the confidence many doctors placed in the echinacea preparation. Fearn also nicely identifies the action of echinacea of the circulatory and lymphatic systems. Modern research has provided a greater understanding of the particulars, but the basic knowledge of these actions was already in the possession of the early American doctor. As Fearn writes, echinacea improves circulation of both blood and lymph, slowly alters the chemistry of the blood, and reduces swelling in lymph glands. The gradual removal of wastes from the body through the stimulation of elimination from skin, kidneys and bowel is also mentioned. In addition, Fearn presents a case wherein the abilities of the plant to retard infection and stimulate the growth of new connective tissues are highlighted. In all of these actions, the basic modes of action accord well with modern findings.

In that same year another famous eclectic physician Finley Ellingwood wrote (and republished in 1983 in the *American Materia Medica, Pharmacology* and *Therapeutics*):

> "The physiological effects are manifested by its action upon the blood, and upon mucous surfaces. The natural secretions are at first augmented, the temperature is then lowered, the pulse is slowed, and the capillary circulation restored.

"It promotes the flow of saliva in an active manner. The warmth and tingling extend down the esophagus to the stomach, but no further unpleasant influence is observed. In a short time diaphoresis is observed, and the continuation of the remedy stimulates the kidneys to increased action. All of the glandular organs seem to feel the stimulating influence, and their functional activity is increased. The stomach is improved in its function, the bowels operate better, and absorption, assimilation, and general nutrition are materially improved. It encourages secretion and excretion, preventing further auto-intoxication, and quickly correcting the influence in the system of any that has occurred. Sallow, pallid and dingy conditions of the skin of the face quickly disappear, and the rosy hue of health is apparent. Anaemic conditions improve with increased nerve tone. . . . It is apparently non-toxic, and to any unpleasant extent non-irritant.

". . . while it equalizes the circulation, it also acts as a sedative to abnormal vascular excitement and lowers the temperature, if this be elevated, while if this be subnormal, the singular effect upon the vital forces conspires toward a restoration of the normal condition."

Like other writers before and after him, Ellingwood lists dozens of ailments for which he had found echinacea beneficial, including boils, carbuncles, abscesses, typhoid fever, puerperal fever, diphtheria, septic fevers, uremic poisoning, post nasal or catarrhal, ulcerations, erysipelas, bed sores, fever sores, bites and stings of poisonous animals, phlebitis, and urethral infection.

Ellingwood is the first eclectic to mention in writing the tonic nature of echinacea, that is, the ability of the plant to normalize cellular processes, no matter which way they depart from normal. This tonic action was discussed the next year by another eclectic doctor whose penchant for laboratory research yielded some remarkable observations about echinacea.

In an article published in 1915,[9] V. von Unruh discusses the cellular physiologic action of echinacea. From this time forward, the science of echinacea would be grounded in scientific observation and manipulation.

"In its therapeutic action, the drug is found to produce direct stimulation of the catabolic processes, increase in the flow of saliva, sweat and urine, increase in glandular activity. It thus antagonizes all septic processes, facilitates the elimination of toxins from the organism, and lastly, it has a destructive effect upon the streptococci, staphylococci, and other pyogenic organisms.

"My own laboratory researches, conducted for a period of over three years, have shown that echinacea increases the phagocytic power of the leucocytes; it effects a shift to the right and normal in the neutrophiles (Arneth count) where a shift to the left had previously obtained. . . . The leucocytes are directly stimulated by echinacea, their activity is increased, the percentage among the different classes of neutrophiles is rendered normal, and phagocytosis is thus raised to its best functioning capacity.

My experiments showed that even with a cell count of bad prognosis the influence of the compound or of echinacea alone will re-establish a normal or nearly normal cell count, thus raising the phagocytic power of the neutrophiles to its possible maximum. Hyper-leukocytosis and leukopenia are directly improved by echinacea; the proportion of white to red cells is rendered normal; the percentage among neutrophiles becomes normal; and phagocytosis is very evident where formerly no sign of it could be detected under the microscope.

". . . I feel free to state that it is: (1) non-toxic; (2) increases appetite and favors assimilation of food; (3) controls night sweats; (4) materially assists in the elimination of toxins from the organism; (5) favorably influences fever, reducing the temperature to normal; (6) increases phagocytosis; (7) destroys tubercle bacilli; (8) effects an arrest of the disease or a clinical cure in cases that are deemed curable at all, in less time than is required by other present-day methods."

Thus, von Unruh observed the effect of echinacea on components of the immune system decades before the immune system became a subject of concern in orthodox medicine. Most importantly he observed the tonic action of this plant. He described conditions in which echinacea increased white blood cell count and conditions under which the herb decreased white blood cell count. He noticed also that echinacea exerted a greater action on phagocytes than directly on pathogens. Thus it tended to increase the body's own natural resistance to infection, not to just kill germs. This idea, still foreign to modern American medicine, was echoed a decade later by an anonymous writer for an eclectic journal:[10]

> "It is not necessary to assume that a remedy must have a direct chemical effect upon bacteria for it to have germ-destroying action. The human body undoubtedly possesses the power to destroy such organisms, not only with the action of the blood corpuscles, but by means that we do not yet understand. A remedy may increase this germ resistance power, without in any way falling into the class of antiseptics. I do not mean to say that Echinacea has a direct anti-septic effect, but rather, that it has a revitalizing action upon those tissues that resist the action of pathogenic bacteria."

Von Unruh's research set the stage for an era of meticulous research on medicinal plants—not just echinacea, but indeed on all herbal agents employed by the early American doctor. Unfortunately, for reasons that will soon become apparent, that research would be played out in Europe, not in America. Before turning to the beginning of the end of the eclectic school of medicine, let us read more about the period of greatest echinacea application. In 1917, J. U. Lloyd wrote *A Treatise on Echinacea*, published by Lloyd Brothers of Cincinnati, Ohio. This pamphlet contained excerpts that comprised the sum total of all contributions made to the *Eclectic Medical Journal* during the period of 1888 to 1901. Space will not permit reprinting all of these here, but two of the more interesting are presented to provide a flavor of not just the state of echinacea research and application during that era, but to demonstrate the state of conventional or "regular" medicine, and the political rivalry that existed between eclectic and regular physicians, a rivalry which could not be reconciled except through an act of Congress.

> "Mr. K weighs nearly two hundred pounds; temperate in all things, and now looks a perfect picture of health. Some ten months ago he was annoyed by boils. He applied to the hospital of the Missouri Pacific Railroad in this city and received the attention of the head of the establishment, whose regularity

would equal that of a country 'schoolma'am.' He was given medicines of all kinds save that necessary to give him relief. The suppurations grew worse, assuming the condition of carbuncles, and of these he had three or four at a time. The surgeon of the establishment cut and slashed these growths after the most approved fashion. This went on for some time until the man became completely discouraged and made up his mind that the trouble would kill him before he got through with it. At this juncture I put him upon echinacea in form of half an ounce of the specific medicine to a four-ounce mixture, a teaspoonful every three hours. No more carbuncles or boils came. Those that he already had dried up and gradually left him. It has now been about two months, and he is entirely free from his former annoyance, and says he believed this medicine saved his life."[11]

"**The Newer Remedies: Echinacea.** Perhaps this remedy is the most important one that has been introduced in recent years into Eclectic medicine. It stands today the best remedy for fluid changes within the body. Remedies which act as this one does, produce changes, or prevent alterations, that we can not explain. Whatever the changes may be, we know that a better condition of the blood and fluids results from its use. It seems to cover the ground ascribed to antiseptics, antiferments, and antizymotics. That it corrects that disturbed balance of the fluids resulting in boils, abscesses, carbuncles, and many pus-forming cellular inflammations, we know by experience."[12]

"A boy twelve years of age was bitten on the upper lip by some poisonous insect and great swelling and pain with an erysipelatous redness, spread up to the eyes. The first physician who saw him thought an ulcerated tooth was the cause of it, and sent him to a dentist, who extracted the one supposed to be the cause of it, but it was sound, and then the pain and swelling continued to grow worse. I was then called, and recognizing it as blood poisoning, made a solution of specific medicine echinacea by adding two drachmas to four ounces of water, and gave a teaspoonful every two hours. There was manifest improvement in a few hours, and complete recovery in three days. . . . I now believe the case would have been sooner over if the doses had been repeated oftener."[13]

One can readily see that in the writings of the eclectics, mild to great disdain is often expressed for the perceived failings of orthodox medicine. The eclectics felt that they had an inside track to wise and effective medicine, that their approach was more considerate of the patient, that health, wellness and healing came from within rather than without, and so forth. Naturally, the regulars felt with equal passion that the orthodox medicine was best, while the homeopaths held that their approach offered the most hope for mankind.

A clear understanding concerning the differences among the three major schools of medicine in nineteenth and early twentieth century America can be found in a tract from this era written by J. M. Scudder about 1885.[14] Although homeopathy played only a tangential role in the history of echinacea, the fates of homeopathy and eclecticism were similar, although it could be argued that the homeopaths fared better in the political fight with the regulars, obtaining in the end some degree of authorization, while the eclectics lost out altogether. In the introduction to his essay, Scudder writes the following:

"It is possible that the time may come when there will be but one practice of medicine, and when there will be but one designation for the followers of the healing art—that of physician. But that time will not come until men have so greatly changed that they will concede freedom of belief and freedom of action to all who may differ with them in belief and practice. So long as it inheres in man to coerce his neighbors to believe and act as he does, so long will there be sects in medicine as there are in religion."

Scudder did not foresee in his day that a time would come when America would possess a state-sanctioned religion of medicine. That idea would have been as repulsive to him as the idea of state religion was to his forefathers. It should be equally repulsive to us. The people of this country have been poorly served by allowing one school of medical thought the privilege of having the legislative dispensation to completely monopolize the modern health care industry.

A short time after Scudder penned his insightful lines, a series of studies on echinacea were carried out by the American Medical Association, i.e., by the regulars. These trials impugned the effectiveness of echinacea and by extension the validity of the entire eclectic movement, and eventually became a significant part of the criteria used by Congress to grant a charter to the AMA but not to the eclectics.

That the AMA would eventually gain the upper hand in American medicine was evident almost from the moment the AMA was founded in 1846. Schisms within medical disciplines were common, as was disenchantment with medical degrees in general. The AMA announced that its major aim was to clean up the profession. Within a short time the AMA adopted a Code of Ethics that barred its members from consulting with homeopaths and eclectics and all others who were not members of the AMA. By the turn of the century, the AMA had effectively instituted a program in most states that forbade the granting of a license to practice medicine to graduates of any medical schools except those sanctioned by the association.

By 1910, the AMA had conducted and published some negative research on echinacea. When their efforts failed to diminish the popularity of the eclectic treatment, they attacked it again in 1920. In his 1923 tract, J. U. Lloyd reviewed the history and status of echinacea in America, looking for the root causes of the "official" disaffection of the AMA. He made the following points:

• The manner in which echinacea was introduced (as a constituent of a 'home-cure remedy') did not endear it to the regular physicians of the day.

• The tendency for the regulars to reject was further compounded by its close association with the eclectics.

• John King, M.D., an "irregular," was responsible for its introduction. However, during the intervening years, Dr. King's reputation as an accomplished investigator increased steadily, so much so that Dr. Charles Rice, Chairman of the Committee of Revision of the Pharmacopeia of the United States, made the following assessment of King's written work: "It constitutes a precious encyclopedia of medical American plants, and their therapeutical uses. It is a very useful work for reference. Its author is as fine a botanist as a judicial observer of therapeutical effects."

• The reputation of echinacea itself suffered from too many inclusions in lay and unprofessional medicinals with questionable therapeutic value.

• In contrast to the hundreds of favorable observations submitted by American physicians, pharmacological evaluation sponsored by the American Medical Association failed to find significant therapeutic worth in echinacea.

• No university professor or standard medical text had commended echinacea.

• Echinacea was not included in the latest revision of the Pharmacopeia of the United States.

• Major medical journals refused to accept echinacea as a legitimate therapeutic agent. Instead several editorials appeared that banned echinacea. Here are a few excerpts from editorial comments made by members of the AMA.

"These absurd claims (referring to label copy on echinacea preparations) of an evidently ignorant man have passed into the more recent proprietary advertising matters and into much of the eclectic writings. Indeed, the seemingly impossible has been attained by even surpassing Meyer's all-but-all-embracing claims.

"It is worth noticing—although it is not surprising—that these far-reaching claims have been made on no better basis than that of clinical trials by unknown men who have not otherwise achieved any general reputation as acute, discriminating and reliable observers. No attempt seems to have been made to verify these claims by accurate scientific methods, clinical or otherwise, although this could very easily have been done.

"In view of the lack of scientific scrutiny of the claims made for it, echinacea is deemed unworthy of further consideration until more reliable evidence is presented in its favor."[15]

"Like many other discarded drugs, it has failed to sustain the reputation given it by enthusiasts years ago; it is now seldom prescribed under its own name. In common with numerous other little-used drugs, it is finding a place in proprietary mixtures, whose manufacturers make use of the early enthusiastic and unverified reports to endow their nostrums with remarkable therapeutic properties."[15]

These accusations by the AMA may remind a few readers of similar remarks being made today by AMA members. Some things never change. In fact the entire eclectic/AMA debate is as timely today as it was then. The eclectics espoused views of medicine that would be enthusiastically accepted by most members of the alternative health movement of modern America, even if some of the particulars would be rejected. The debate with orthodox medicine, its stranglehold on health care, predicaments with insurance acceptance, patent issues and so forth recapitulate the eclectic dilemma in all its important aspects. The eclectics were driven out of business. Then and now, alternative health care is not allowed to get a foothold.

Some regular physicians during the eclectic/regular debates supported the use of echinacea. However, throughout the 1920s and much of the 1930s, editorials and articles in peer-review medical journals recognized the widespread acceptance of echinacea despite the "official" party line espoused by the AMA. Years later in the 1990s, echinacea would once again come to the forefront of popularity and controversy.

An AMA-sponsored study on echinacea was carried out in the Government Laboratory, Washington, D.C., in 1920, by James F. Couch and Leigh T. Giltner. This study, entitled "An experimental study of echinacea therapy," investigated the effects of several echinacea preparations in guinea pigs infected with tetanus, septicemia, anthrax, dried powdered rattlesnake venom, botulism, tuberculosis, and trypanosomiasis. Their conclusion:

> "In no one of the diseases treated with Echinacea preparations was any evidence obtained to show that the plant exerts any influence upon the course of infectious process under laboratory conditions." Further they state that, "It does not appear, therefore, that the preparations of Echinacea are of value in the treatment of disease produced by microorganisms and their toxic products."[17]

Notice how this last statement generalizes the inactivity of echinacea from a group of highly toxic substances to the whole universe of mircroorganisms, including those of less deadly nature that cause sore throats, colds, influenza, skin infections, herpes, and so forth.

The inclusion of botulism and tetanus in this study is questionable from the start, since echinacea was not typically used in either of these two situations. Other problems with the interpretations of the results obtained by Couch and Giltner were discussed the next year by James H. Beal in the *American Journal of Pharmacy*,[18] in which he pointed out that in almost every case, the results could be interpreted to show that echinacea did indeed have some value in the course of the infection, i.e., there was a distinct tendency for treated animals to outlive non-treated animals.

Perhaps a longer time-course in the study would have produced statistically significant results. In spite of Beal's appeal, the AMA's Council on Pharmacy and Chemistry rejected echinacea on the grounds of insufficient evidence for therapeutic efficacy, the same grounds they would use from that time until the present to reject botanical agents brought forward from any quarter except the American pharmaceutical conglomerate.

To the credit of the practicing American doctor, the publication of Couch and Giltner's work did little to discourage the therapeutic use of echinacea. Lloyd Brothers' response to the study was to suspend all advertising of echinacea for one year following publication of the study. During that year, they sent out survey cards to hundreds of physicians requesting them to share their experience with echinacea preparations in their individual practices. They received over 700 responses. By far the majority of physicians, many of whom were "regular" M.D.s, responded that they used echinacea for septic, or infectious, conditions. Both internal and external infections were treated. The terms *blood poisoning, blood dyscrasias* and *depraved blood* occur dozens of times in the responses. Textual comments indicate that early American physicians believed that most infectious conditions affected the blood, either by imparting unwholesome qualities to it, or by destroying its very fabric. Experience with snake and insect bites certainly substantiated this view. Many doctors reported using echinacea in the treatment of snakebite, thus confirming Meyer's original thesis.

The term *alterative* also appears frequently in the survey. An alterative was an agent believed to help restore health to the blood by gently altering its characteristics from negative to positive. A few physicians recognized this as a tonic function and so indicated in their responses. Among the specific infections mentioned, typhoid stands out. This was one of the commonest and most deadly of frontier infections, and agents for use in its treatment were highly prized by the doctor. Other specific infections mentioned in the survey results were peritonitis, syphilis, diphtheria, puerperal fever, tonsillitis, scarlet fever, spotted fever, ptomaine poisoning and ulcers. External conditions appeared very often in the survey, including sores, wounds, surgical wounds, punctures, eye infections, erysipelas, eruptions, boils, bites, pain, gangrene and ringworm.

In summary the picture that emerges from this rather extensive survey shows that both "regular" and "irregular" doctors were employing echinacea in the early 1900's as an antiseptic, anti-infectious, alterative and tonic substance with few equals. In fact, Lloyd Brothers presented data showing that by 1921–22, echinacea was outselling the next highest selling botanical preparation by more than two to one.

In the year 1927, while Lloyd was desperately trying to underscore the legitimacy of echinacea, and the AMA was pompously dismissing the substance, other eclectic physicians wrote material that was both good and bad, from a political point of view.

By 1930, the areas for which echinacea was deemed suitable had stabilized somewhat. In *A Handy Reference Book*,[19] J. S. Niederkorn discusses the application of echinacea for several purposes individually. These areas are: blood; diarrhea and dysentery; fevers; mammary gland infection; mouth sores; rheumatism; skin and tissue; stomach and intestines.

Trying to shore up the reputation of echinacea occupied the time and effort of several eclectics during the late 1920s and most of the 1930s. Among these were S. H. Cutler and L. Fellow. In 1931 they published a review of echinacea research and clinical experience that broadened the understanding of the plant and referenced some of the more credible case histories.[20]

At this point, the AMA stranglehold tightened considerably. Almost overnight, the eclectic movement stopped. The regulars had finally won the long struggle. Their monopoly was complete (except for a handful of homeopaths that managed through astute political positioning to obtain a special charter under a "grandfather" provision). All writing on echinacea ceased abruptly in 1937 in the medical literature and no mention of echinacea has been printed since in the United States. Echinacea went from a position of high visibility to total obscurity in this country in a period of time so short it boggles the mind.

The story of echinacea might have ended in the late 1930s were it not for a very lucky occurrence. A German firm, intrigued by what was happening with echinacea in the United States, requested a quantity of seed from the Lloyd brothers. German interest in echinacea led to a general European interest in the plant, and over the next 60 years the popularity of echinacea, both as a favorite immunotonic, and as a subject of research, grew ever more rapidly.

It wasn't until the 1970's that echinacea was reintroduced to Americans from European manufacturers. As the encapsulated herb market in general gained in popularity during that decade, echinacea became established as a major herb in the "new" materia medica. The irony is that this most important native North American plant may have been lost to us if it hadn't been for the work of Europeans that resulted from a chance delivery of seed from Lloyd Brothers. Although America is still not doing any scientific research on echinacea, at least we are in a position to take advantage of the work our European brothers are doing.

ECHINACEA RESEARCH AND APPLICATIONS

In the following sections we will review some of the pertinent research on echinacea and suggest practical ways echinacea may be used to realize its full healing potential.

Echinacea and the Skin/Connective Tissue

Whether skin damage results from the presence of infection or is due to injury, echinacea can aid in the healing of such damage. This knowledge has been around since the beginning of echinacea's history, but recent research has helped us understand the mechanisms involved.

One of the main actions of echinacea is to inhibit a particular enzyme that is involved in weakening the structure of connective tissue in the presence of certain microorganisms. The enzyme is called hyaluronidase and is part of the hyaluronidase system. It affects the activity of a part of connective tissue ground substance known as hyaluronic acid (HA). HA acts as a barrier to pathogens. Under certain conditions, however, HA is weakened through a conspiracy between hyaluronidase and these pathogens to reduce the viscosity, or integrity, of HA.

This process can be compared to the degradation of a bowl of jello. Once the integrity of connective tissues has been compromised by the pathogen/hyaluronidase activity, infectious organisms gain easy access to the deeper cells and tissues of the skin and body, including blood vessels and lymphatic tissues, where they create pockets of infection. Substances in echinacea inhibit hyaluronidase and thereby stabilize connective tissues and strengthen the body's first line of defense against infection.[1-3] This action has important consequences for accelerating the healing process after trauma to skin or other connective tissues. Daily consumption of small amounts of whole, dried, encapsulated echinacea is important for improving our defensive barriers to germs that assault us in the environment.

The anti-hyaluronidase action of echinacea has also been implicated in the regeneration of connective tissue (granulation) destroyed during infection or as the result of injury. Basically, echinacea stimulates fibroblasts to greater effort in producing hyaluronic acid and repairing injured tissue. New fibrocytes appear more rapidly and on a larger scale, and are more quickly recruited in the formation of new tissue, primarily mucopolysaccharides, in the mesoderm layer of the skin. Enhanced activity in the mesoderm leads to increased production of all types of connective tissue, as well as bone marrow, blood and lymph.[4-7]

Skin Wounds

The use of echinacea extracts and fresh poultices in wound healing by the eclectics was certainly widespread and has persisted, primarily in Europe, in the decades following their demise. Some research in this area has been productive. Perhaps the most extensive study of its kind was performed by the German P. Viehmann in 1978. He reported a 91.5% success rate in healing wounds with a topical echinacin ointment.[8] Other studies have found topical and oral applications of echinacea extracts effective in treating first-, second- and third-degree burns, skin injuries and sports-related abrasions.[9] In a report of one study, the author described in great detail how echinacea ointment helped to clean and heal wounds, reduce the risk of secondary infections and relieve pain and exerted a dramatic effect on the formation of new granulation tissue and epidermis without concomitant scarring.[10] In an animal study, echinacea ointment was applied to skin wounds in guinea pigs and compared to treatment with placebo; the results showed much more rapid healing in treated animals.[11] Topical dressings for skin injuries can be prepared from fresh echinacea roots and tops, or can be purchased from health food stores. A simple recipe for an ointment is given later in this book.

Animal Bites

Topical and internal applications of echinacea have been popular in the treatment of bites and stings from animals, insects, spiders and snakes. Everything from rattlesnake bites and black widow bites to mosquito and flea bites can be treated with the plant. Modern research in this area is lacking, but there is certainly no dearth of modern testimonials. People quickly learn that the application of echinacea directly into a stricken area exerts an immediate positive effect on the course of the problem, resulting in decreased pain, accelerated healing and a cessation to any spreading of toxin that would otherwise occur. Taking it internally at the same time as external treatment also seems to improve the healing power of the plant. In spite of the successful use of echinacea for bites, as reported by numerous individuals, the lack of good scientifically controlled trials in this area should serve as a caution to not forego medical treatment in the case of a serious or life-threatening encounter with animal venom. It should also be noted that the consumption of excessive amounts of echinacea during an acute infection from a venomous source will almost certainly invoke a healing crisis involving fever.

Skin Disease

A great deal of research has been done on the ability of echinacea to affect the course of skin disease. For example, German scientists have reported that echinacea extracts produce a rapid and complete restoration of skin tissue following infection. Some authors attribute the effect to the acceleration of phagocytosis rates in the area of the infection.[12] In a rather extensive study, a team of scientists reported extremely good results in treating a wide variety of skin diseases using an echinacea salve. Out of 4,598 patients, a full 85.5% responded successfully to the treatment. These patients presented with all kinds of abscesses, wounds and ulcerated conditions. Some suffered from dermatitis and folliculitis, and dozens suffered from many kinds of inflammatory skin conditions.[13] These kinds of results have been obtained by other researchers in similar and other afflictions, including pemphigus vulgaris,[14] psoriasis,[15,16] eczema,[17] herpes simplex,[18] and others.[19]

It is apparent from the research, as well as from the extensive eclectic literature on this subject, that echinacea application can significantly reduce infection and accelerate the growth of new tissue. The form of administration may be important. Orally, the effect is much slower than topically, and the most effective route appears to be by injection. Because the injectable form of echinacea is illegal in this country (being an unapproved drug), we must make do with ointments and poultices prepared from fresh plant material. These latter forms are still effective and will prove extremely useful in most cases, especially if combined with other tissue healing herbs such as lapacho, comfrey and horsetail.

ECHINACEA AND THE IMMUNE SYSTEM

Many of the actions of echinacea described above apply equally to its actions on the immune system. There is a great deal of overlap between the immune system and the musculo-skeletal system and many of the physiological processes that protect the skin are really components of the immune system. The skin is often viewed as the first line of defense against invading microorganisms and maintaining its integrity is a major task of the immune system. In addition to improving the protective ability of the skin, however, echinacea exerts dozens of other important influences on our immune processes.

Many echinacea extracts show strong stimulating effects on the immune system, while other extracts seem to be able to suppress immune function. Still other extracts, as well as the whole plant, exert a tonic effect, i.e., they can either lower or raise immune function depending on the changing needs of the body. Extracting principles from whole plant material runs the risk of leaving behind certain constituents that lend the herb this balancing action. Only extracts that are carefully pre-pared so as to retain all active fractions of the plant retain the tonic action. While many suppliers of echinacea claim full spectrum activity for their extracts, in reality very few do any kind of clinical research to validate this claim.

Echinacea as an Immunotonic

The immunotonic action of echinacea is a good example of plant materials helping the body help itself. By supplying the nutrients required by the immune system to stay healthy, echinacea may be considered a primary immune system agent. As a tonic, echinacea can both increase and decrease immune system activity. Thus, it can raise white blood cell count and activity, or it may lower these parame-ters. This means that it must contain substances that act in opposition to one another. An extract that leaves one group of constituents behind, or weakens it, will lack the tonic activity. The tonic concept also demands that the body be able to recognize and utilize one group of constituents while ignoring the other. In the case of echinacea, as with all proven tonics, these conditions are fulfilled. The plant does contain opposite acting, or *bidirectional,* constituents and the body is able to recognize which to use. (For a complete discussion of bidirectionality and herbal tonics, the reader is referred to *Herbal Tonic Therapies,* Keats Publishing, 1993.)

While the term "white blood cell" is generally used to describe the entire immune system package, the system is actually composed of numerous substances and has been the subject of extensive cataloging. There are two important aspects of immune function, *humoral immunity* and *cell-mediated immunity.* Each of these is affected dramatically by echinacea. Humoral immunity involves the action of antibodies, complement and B-cells, while cell-mediated immunity depends on T-cells. We can also classify certain cells, such as macrophages, neutrophils and natural killer cells as *nonspecific effector cells.* Additionally, we can classify certain cells as *phagocytes,* such as neutrophils and eosinophils. Still another grouping of immune system components is possible. The *granulocyte* category includes neutrophils, eosinophils, basophils and mast cells. All of these components interact with one another, and classification schemes are only meaningful as a way of organizing certain processes into readily understandable chunks. We will not attempt an exhaustive review of all of the processes in this book, and our discussion of echinacea may leap from one area to another without considering any organizational scheme. The reader will discover, however, that echinacea affects almost every known immune process to one extent or another.

Research on echinacea's role in immune functioning began with the studies of von Unruh, discussed earlier in this book. Even at that early date, he was able to describe the tonic action of echinacea on white blood cell activity. With the demise of the Eclectic Medical Association in the 1930s, all American research on echinacea ended. Research began again following World War II in the 1950s in Germany. The Germans had obtained seed of *Echinacea purpurea* from the Lloyd Brothers, and had been cultivating it for many years. They had observed many of the same clinical results as the Americans had, and determined that it should be the subject of extensive clinical investigation. The result was the publication of dozens of research papers on the therapeutic action of this plant. As mentioned before, most of this research utilized preparations made from the flowers and leaves of the plant, while Americans had been using the roots. In addition, some German preparations were administered via injection, a route of administration rarely used in America. Finally, whereas Americans had been using E. angustifolia, the Germans had obtained the E. purpurea seed by mistake. As a result of these differences, one would expect the research results of European scientists to deviate somewhat from the observations of American eclectics. That such deviations were seldom observed attests to the strength of therapeutic activity in all parts of these two species of echinacea, independent of mode of preparation or route of administration.

Interestingly, modern research, using more sophisticated equipment, has validated some of von Unruh's work. In one study, Echinacin stimulated an increase in leukocyte production following radiation therapy. Leukocytes steadily increased for three hours following injection, and gradually returned to normal levels, suggesting a tonic action at work.[20] A certain portion of this work has suggested that persons with severely weakened immune systems will not respond to echinacea treatment as readily as more healthy individuals. This observation indicates that you should not wait too long before initiating treatment with echinacea. Powdered, encapsulated echinacea exerts a tonic effect and may be consumed regularly throughout the year without fear of overdosage or habituation. Thus, the practice of regular echinacea consumption should help maintain the immune system in a state of health at all times and dramatically improve the body's ability to resist invasion by noxious microorganisms.

By far the greatest amount of research on echinacea has examined its ability to increase general cellular immunity. Space will not allow a complete review here, but excellent reviews are available elsewhere.[21-24] Purified polysaccharides from echinacea exert a strong activation on the macrophage-mediated defense system. Macrophages are structures in the immune system that initiate the destruction of harmful microorganisms and pathogens that cause bacterial and viral infections and cancer. Echinacea activates the macrophage directly, as well as indirectly through a stimulatory effect on T-cells. Activated macrophages not only attack pathogens, they also initiate other immune responses through the production and secretion of interleukin-1 and B lymphocytes.[25,26] Although we will discuss the antimicrobial action of echinacea separately, it should be noted here that this action is probably partly the result of the stimulation of phagocytosis.[27] Among the afflictions studied in European laboratories and clinics and successfully treated with echinacea are meningitis, psoriasis, whooping cough, ear infections, tuberculosis, tonsillitis, bronchitis, colds, flus and several kinds of wounds, as listed earlier.

In an important series of experiments by German investigators it was found, among other findings, that polysaccharides in echinacea increased T-cell activity by 20 to 30 percent more than control drugs known to possess strong T-cell stimulating properties.[28,29] Other researchers have found what they consider better results using lipophilic (non-polysaccharide) fractions of the plant.[30] In fact, it appears that almost all fractions of the plant are capable of enhancing general immunity to one degree or another.

Results such as these have both elucidated the action of echinacea and partially confused the issues surrounding its practical application. Because most echinacea research employs *extracts* of the plant, it is possible that some of the tonic nature of the plant is often compromised. The production of echinacea extracts has become big business both overseas and in this country. As the technology increases, the extracts become increasingly pure, i.e., more of the plant is left behind. Very few manufacturers, however, have the ability to produce an extract that is truly full-spectrum, i.e., one that retains all of the activity of the parent plant. Many extracts are advertised as being full-spectrum, but probably are not. With better extract technology but lack of control standards to insure full-spectrum activity, the market becomes cluttered with non-tonic extracts. Therefore, in both controlled research using extracts and in uncontrolled clinical settings, scientists and herbalists have observed that long-term use actually weakens general immune responsiveness. Extracts that do this should therefore only be used intermittently, as needed. We maintain, however, that the tonic nature of the whole plant and true full-spectrum extracts prevent problems due to regular usage, and that they in fact help to keep the immune system in proper balance at all times.

The therapeutic action of echinacea on the immune system results in a certain amount of housecleaning. Increased phagocytosis results in the degradation of wastes, toxins, pathogens and other foreign material floating around in the blood and lymph. The purification of the circulatory and lymphatic systems is what the herbalists have meant by the term "blood purification." The "old" term for waste-laden blood was sepsis, in its strongest sense a kind of blood poisoning. Today we know that sepsis can be avoided by consuming immunotonics such as echinacea. As you review many of the quotes in previous pages you will note how often the idea of blood purification arises. Though it may seem like an antiquated concept, it is directly in line with what is known about immunological processes and is at the forefront of modern medicinal notions. The lymph system was only vaguely understood until recently. Now we know that it is of critical importance in ridding the body of waste. Echinacea undoubtedly enhances the action of this system and exerts much of its purification/cleansing action through this means.

Allergies

In most cases, consumption of echinacea leads to an increase in white blood cell activity. However, whole plant material or a good full-spectrum extract can exert certain actions that could be classified as immunosuppressive, i.e., they actually reduce immune responsiveness. The body's first response to the presence of an allergen is to type it and memorize it and file this information away for future reference. The physiological response is usually very small. The next time the allergen shows up, however, the body initiates efforts to get rid of it. This immune response can get out of hand, becoming much too extreme for the limited amount of allergen at hand. This is the allergic response. Allergic symptoms arise when basophils and mast cells erupt in response to the allergen and discharge their content of histamine, bradykinin and other substances into the blood. Echinacea reduces this response by stabilizing the mast cell and increasing its ability to resist breakage in the presence of allergens. The practical result is a dramatic reduction in allergic symptoms—good news for all of us. This ability of a tonic substance to both augment and suppress immune response is not shared by any known drug and is a good reason to prefer herbal tonic materials over the non-tonic herbals and the synthetic drugs.

Echinacea as an Immunostimulant
    The immunostimulant function of echinacea is found in virtually all different kinds of echinacea preparations. Even when the immunosuppressive fractions of the plant have been discarded in the extractive process, the immunostimulating action remains and may be potentiated through the preparation of concentrated extracts. These extracts are ideal for use in the treatment of acute infections of all kinds. Even though you may be consuming a whole, powdered and encapsulated preparation of echinacea on a regular basis, your immune system may still be overcome by the presence of a particularly nasty germ. The throat is usually the first part of the body to encounter and succumb to such infections. When that happens, there is nothing better than a powerful echinacea extract to knock the infection out in a hurry. A dropperful in the back of the throat works wonders. The earlier you apply the treatment, the better will be the results.
    Research on the immunostimulating action of echinacea has shown that it does in fact promote the production and action of antibodies, complement and B-cells, though sometimes only weakly. The complement system is composed of substances that latch onto invaders and signal other components of the immune system to come and destroy them. At least one of the critical factors in the complement system has been shown to be favorably influenced by echinacea. This substance is called *properdin* and is the substance that actually initiates the complement cascade.[31]

ANTIVIRAL ACTION

Finding effective antiviral substances that are not equally toxic to normal cells has been one of the great challenges of medical science. Intriguing research with echinacea suggests that this plant may be one of the more effective antiviral compounds that is also safe to use at effective dosage levels. Several different fractions of the plant have been studied; some work better than others. An early study found that a simple extract had to be combined with a dextran molecule in order to be effective.[32] Later, another researcher discovered that in the petri dish environment, cells had to be pre-treated with an echinacea extract in order to afford protection against various viruses. Interestingly, he found that both ethanol and aqueous extracts were about equally effective, and were even more effective when combined.[33] This study was replicated a couple of years later by Wacker and Hilbig with similar results. This time it was found that pretreatment resulted in 24 to 48 hour protection against influenza virus, herpes, and vesicular stomatitis (canker sore) viruses. These results resembled those obtained with interferon (the only known endogenous antiviral substance). The researchers suggested that echinacea stimulates T-cell lymphocytes which, in turn, produce interferon, or alternatively, it acts through cell surface chemistry, perhaps involving hyaluronidase.[34] This hypothesis has been disputed by other investigators who maintain that a more parsimonious explanation has echinacea actively competing with viruses for receptor sites on cell membrane surfaces.[35] The idea that echinacea stimulates T-lymphocytes has also been disputed. Finally, it was noted that the fresh juice of the whole plant was up to 30 percent more effective than either the water or methanol extracts, and that whole plant juice was more effective than the fresh juice of any isolated part of the plant.

These results mean that people who are consuming echinacea in any form, but especially fresh whole plant, can expect some degree of protection against viral organisms. However, more research is required before we will understand the precise method of action. Incidentally, fresh juice of the whole plant is obtained by expression; this requires exposing the material to considerable pressure. Presses made from hydraulic car jacks can be effective, if commercial presses are beyond your budget. Be sure to maintain good sanitary conditions at all times.

ANTIFUNGAL ACTION

Echinacea has been found effective against at least one common yeast, *Candida albicans*. This yeast is the main pathogen responsible for vaginal yeast infection and has been the topic of a great deal of interest by scientist and layperson alike. Normal treatment for this condition involves the use of antibiotics and antifungal drugs which unfortunately can so overpower the immune system that secondary infections such as vaginitis and urinary tract infection may result. Echinacea preparations, both external and internal, may be a viable alternative to the drug approach. In one study, scientists administered Echinacin either as a liquid internally or as an i.v. injection in conjunction with a standard antifungal agent. After several weeks the echinacea groups were compared to control subjects who received just the antifungal treatment. Regardless of route of administration, the echinacea treatment produced better results than controls and resulted in significantly fewer recurrences of the infection.[36] The implication of this study is that if you have trouble with recurrent vaginal yeast infections, you should try adding a strong echinacea extract to your treatment regimen. You may experience fewer infections of shorter duration.

ANTIBIOTIC ACTION

Surprisingly, the direct antibiotic activity of the echinacea preparations most often studied in European labs has been found to be only modest in strength. A weak action against both staph and strep bacteria has been noted using a glycoside (echinoside) preparation.[37,38] It has been found, however, that another constituent, echinacin, may be more effective than cortisone. For example, streptococcal infection spreads rapidly in guinea pigs pretreated with cortisone, but is contained by the echinacin. It has also been found that 0.04 ml of fresh plant of echinacea extract possesses a hyaluronidase inhibitory action equal to 1 mg of cortisone.[39-41]

In order to take advantage of the antibiotic action of echinacea, we recommend that you use a poultice of fresh root or plant for external applications, and that you obtain and consume a strong fresh extract (you can make your own as described later in this book).

THE RESPIRATORY SYSTEM

Perhaps the most widespread applications of echinacea today are to prevent and treat respiratory diseases such as colds, influenza, tonsillitis, otitis media, whooping cough and other bronchial ailments. Throughout the world, echinacea has gained a reputation for being one of the most effective treatments for these conditions. There is a great deal of research to support these uses.[42-47] Most of the research was conducted in Europe where the route of administration usually employed was the injectable form. However, it has become generally accepted that orally administered echinacea preparations are about as effective as the injected, though sometimes considerably slower in their action. In this country we do not have access to echinacea injections, but the sophistication of many of the preparations that are available makes therapy with echinacea a viable enterprise. Most practitioners agree that the earlier in an infection that echinacea is employed the greater are its chances for success. In fact, the usefulness of echinacea in treating a common cold is greatly reduced once full blown symptoms are present. Hence, you are advised to consume whole, powdered, encapsulated echinacea on a daily basis both before and during the cold and flu season, and to begin taking a concentrated liquid extract at the earliest sign that you may be getting sick.

ARTHRITIS AND INFLAMMATION

A German patent revealed the presence of two factors in echinacea, called *factor A* and *factor B*. Factor A caused a stress response accompanied by fever, while factor B exhibited an antihyaluronidase action. The two factors appeared to be in opposition, as one would expect from a tonic.[48] Factor B was effective in improving the wound healing process. It helped in the production of fibrous scar tissue in the wound. Some researchers suggest that the active principles in echinacea extracts combine with hyaluronic acid to produce a complex that is resistant to attack by hyaluronidase and that both restricts the diffusion of viruses and other microorganisms in the wound and facilitates the regeneration of fibrous connective tissues.[49,50]

Researchers investigating the anti-inflammatory properties of echinacea through the standard carrageenan and croton oil tests have found that echinacea B extracts significantly prevent the inflammation and swelling associated with these tests.[51]

On the practical level, it is not always wise to consume anti-inflammatory agents. Sometimes it is better to let the inflammation run its course. However, in the case of inflammatory joint disease, such as arthritis, or when an infectious inflammation is lingering for an extended period of time, it is best to reduce the inflammation as much as possible. Owing to its tonic nature, echinacea can enhance the inflammatory response to acute infections, and can inhibit the chronic inflammatory response as well. In the clinical setting, echinacea extract exhibits an anti-inflammatory effect equal to about half that from cortisone and prednisone in polyarthritic patients, and is thus well-suited for this application, since the steroids are a poor choice due to their side effects.[52] In addition, echinacea exhibits no side effects, and a good whole-plant extract would be expected to possess the tonic action we have often mentioned in this book. The anti-arthritic effect of echinacea extracts has been established in other studies also.[53,54]

CANCER

Echinacea extracts sometimes possess a strong cytotoxic activity against certain tumor cells. USDA researchers discovered a tumor-inhibiting principle, an oncolytic lipid-soluble hydrocarbon, in the essential oil of echinacea that inhibited Walker's carcinosarcoma and lymphocytic leukemia.[55] Anti-tumor activity has been noted by others as well.[56] The mode of action of echinacea against cancer cells is not clear but probably does not involve a direct cytotoxic action. Rather, echinacea probably enhances the activity of the body's own anti-cancer cells, such as natural killer cells and macrophages (although there is some question about the ability of echinacea to stimulate natural killer cells).[57] Persons desiring to prevent or inhibit cancer would do well to include echinacea in their treatment regimen, but should not rely exclusively on this plant.

SUMMARY OF RESEARCH APPLICATIONS

Over a span of about 30 years, German researchers have been able to explore and document several of the most fundamental properties of echinacea. However, almost all of this research was done on a water extract of the flowering tops of the plant. The only other form of the plant used during this time was a combination containing echinacea, wild indigo and thuja; thus, while the preparation showed good therapeutic properties, it was impossible to determine what contribution echinacea alone made to the observed outcomes. The water extract was (and still is) known as *Echinacin*. The combination is called *Esberitox*. Echinacin is typically administered intravenously, although a small amount of research suggests the oral route of administration is as effective as the i.v. route, though much slower in its effects.

Clinical experience with echinacea in recent years can therefore be roughly divided into two categories. The first is research, ranging in quality from poor to very good, carried out primarily in Europe, and reported in a variety of medical journals. The second is work done in the United States and Canada by a variety of clinical herbalists, chiropractors and naturopaths, published nowhere and typically lacking even the most rudimentary of control procedures. The first category utilized Echinacin almost exclusively (the water extract of flowering tops), administered most often intravenously or via intramuscular injections. The second category utilized a very uneven variety of preparations, including tinctures, fluid extracts, capsules, tablets, teas, whole root, fresh, dried, etc., all taken orally. Many of these were products personally prepared by the practitioner. Other preparations were proprietary products. Roots, stems and flowering tops, singly or in combination, may have been used.

Given the limited scope of European research and the uncontrolled, helter-skelter nature of the American work, what are we to make of the observations of the relative groups? At this point it may be most useful to simply list the various conditions that have been successfully treated, realizing the list is probably not complete, and the range of applications of echinacea is as broad as the number of ailments and problems that could be impacted by enhanced immune system functioning:

• Systemic infections, including cellulitis, colds, flus, etc. Increases specific and nonspecific immune system activities.

• Wounds of all kinds, including, ulcers, sports injuries, burns, lacerations, gun shot wounds, etc. Reduces chance of infection, speeds repair of injured tissues.

• Skin diseases, including impetigo, eczema, folliculitis, dermatitis, herpes, frostbite, chilblains. Speeds healing and regeneration of connective tissue, reduces pain and inflammation.

• Specific infections, including upper respiratory tract infections, tonsillitis, pertussis, bronchitis, gingivitis; candidiasis and other gynecological infections; prostatitis. Inhibits specific microorganisms, accelerates repair processes, stimulates general immune processes. Use of topical creams for candidiasis effective.

• Inflammatory disease, especially rheumatism and arthritis.

• Allergies. Stabilizes basophils and mast cells.

HOW TO GROW YOUR OWN ECHINACEA

Everyone should know how to grow echinacea, even if they don't want to do it at the present time. Freshly grown echinacea is probably a more reliable source of active material than commercial products.

Echinacea tolerates a wide range of conditions, thrives on abuse, and is drought resistant. In addition, disease is not a big problem. *E. purpurea* is thought to be easier to grow than *E. angustifolia*, but neither one is a big problem. The main difference is that *E. angustifolia* requires direct sun, while *E. purpurea* requires partial shade. Both require good drainage, this being more critical for *E. angustifolia*.

Soil. Use light, stone-free soil, with humus. It should hold water, but allow good drainage. Echinacea roots do not thrive in standing water. Keep weed free.

Fertilizer. Before planting: use potash, preferably obtained from wood ash; phosphate, such as bone meal or from rock. After planting: use nitrogen occasionally.

Propagating. There are three main ways to propagate echinacea, discussed individually below.

    1. **From seed.** Seed is readily available from catalogs and nurseries. It may be sowed directly into the ground, or stratified. It is highly recommended that *E. angustifolia* be stratified, and the stratification of *E. purpurea* will also increase the chances of successful germination. (Stratification techniques are discussed below.) Seed may be sowed directly in the garden any time of year, but the fall is by far the best time. Protect seed with straw mulch during winter months. Following stratification, wash seeds to remove sand, and germinate the seed either in flats indoors or out-

side on beds of good soil. Use a good sprouting mixture, or a mix that contains ⅓ sand, ⅓ peat and ⅓ sterile potting soil. Do not bury the seed in the soil; simply place on top and tamp down on soil surface. Germinate for about two weeks, but there is no need to rush transplanting the seedlings.

2. **By dividing.** A good way to increase your crop is to divide the roots and crowns of existing plants in the spring or fall (best). Separating two to three inches of roots with the crown is thought to be the best procedure. You should be able to obtain two to seven buds from one crown. These can be planted directly in a spot with appropriate soil. A plant should be at least two years old before it can be safely divided. Obtaining roots and crowns from a friend is a good way to start a crop.

3. **By purchasing plants.** Buy from mail order catalogues and local nurseries potted echinacea plants that can be planted directly in the garden. If all you want are a few good plants, this is undoubtedly the easiest way to get started.

Planting. When ready, set the seedlings in beds one to two feet apart with perlite and a good general soil mixture. The seedlings should be at least six to seven weeks old. Keep moist. Seedlings may be set out in the fall or in the spring, but most experts agree that fall is by far the best time, late October or early November. If you stratify the seed by placing it in moist sand outside during the winter, you will be forced to transplant seedlings in the spring. Don't expect *E. angustifolia* to flower until the third year; *E. purpurea* may flower during the first year, but usually waits until the second year to flower.

Harvesting. Harvest in the fall. The flowering tops and stems of echinacea may be harvested from the first year that flowers appear. Three- to four-year-old roots may be harvested. Roots should be cleaned and dried under low forced heat or outside in the shade. Fresh juice may be expressed from fresh roots.

The seed may be harvested in the fall, after the stalks turn brown. Cut whole heads and dry at 35 degrees C. Thresh out the seed. It may be stored for several years in the refrigerator.

Stratification. Stratification increases the yield seed significantly. This is important only if you are trying to raise a large crop. Seed may be stratified indoors or outdoors.

1. **Indoors:** Stratify by placing seed in moist, but not wet, sand and storing in the refrigerator in a plastic bag for 90 to 160 days.

2. **Outdoors:** The seed is prepared as in indoor stratifying, using a mix of sand and peat, and is then placed outside over the winter, covered with a mesh screen.

HOW TO MAKE YOUR OWN EXTRACT

There is some controversy about what kind of echinacea extract is best. The debate revolves around at least three issues: species, part and menstruum. The question of species may be easily resolved by the layman growing his own: Use *E. angustifolia* or *E. purpurea.* The question of what part of the plant to use is a little more difficult to answer. Echinacin, the popular German product, is made solely from the flowering tops. However, the roots are used in dozens of other proprietary products for which great efficacy is claimed. A possible practical solution to this problem is to prepare and use both parts of the plant and decide for yourself which is most suitable for your own applications. Combine both together as a third, perhaps best, alternative.

The third question is the most troublesome for the novice: what medium (menstruum) is best to prepare an echinacea extract? Your choices are as follows: water; ethanol; water plus ethanol in equal proportions; high water, low ethanol; low water, high ethanol; vinegar or glycerine. If you choose not to extract at all, you may chew the fresh or dried plant parts directly.

Assuming you wish to extract, it is my opinion that a cold or hot water extract of fresh or dried plant may be used. A hot water extract of the flowering tops and stems is a simple tea. A hot water extract of the roots is prepared by steeping the roots in near-boiling hot water for 20 to 30 minutes before consuming.

Water extracts contain no preservative and must be discarded in a matter of hours following preparation if not entirely consumed. Preparations for storage must contain a preservative. This is usually alcohol. Vinegar and glycerine extracts do not contain alcohol; their shelf life is longer than water extracts, but shorter than alcohol, several weeks or a few months at best.

A convenient way to obtain a menstruum of both alcohol and water is to use vodka, gin or other alcoholic product. A ratio of water to alcohol of 60:40, or 50:50 is commonly used although you may want to try other ratios. An alternative to prepared products like vodka is to acquire Everclear and distilled water and mix your own. Lloyd felt that a 69 percent alcohol menstruum was best. Once the menstruum has been acquired, place a few ounces of echinacea in a mason jar, cover with menstruum, close lid, shake, and set aside for two weeks, shaking the jar a couple of times each day. Then, after two weeks, strain and press out as much liquid from the plant material as possible (a tourniquet made with a cloth diaper and a stick is a good way to press out the fluid). Discard remaining plant material. This simple extract of root or flowering tops and stems, or both, should be effective (a tingling sensation on the tongue is a simple indicator of probable therapeutic effectiveness) and will store for long periods. Avoid exposure to heat and direct sunlight.

Sometimes a fourth problem is encountered: is fresh plant or dried plant best? Many commercial echinacea products are encapsulated ground dried echinacea. These capsules are swallowed. The advantage to the ground whole plant is that it is not an extract. It is the whole plant material. Whole plant may possess greater tonic action than an extract. The disadvantage is lack of research data on such preparations. Perhaps the use of a combination of extract and whole plant would be the wisest course of action. I believe that encapsulated powdered echinacea is most appropriate for daily use as a tonic to help keep the immune system in a state of balance, but that an extract is more suitable in case of acute infection, used for short periods of time only.

Dried material may be extracted also. Whether you dry the plant yourself, or purchase it already dried, follow the same procedures for extracting as used for fresh material.

Making your own ointment is also an easy process, though you will no doubt do some experimentation on your own to develop just the right consistency. You will need: 2 to 3 cups of dried echinacea stems, flowering tops and/or root; 2 cups distilled water; 1 cup olive oil; 1 to 2 ounces of beeswax; a few drops of essential oil for fragrance; a double boiler; spoon; strainer; storage jar, preferrably dark glass; tincture of Benzoin (from drugstore). Bring water to boil, add herbs and boil down to ½ cup. Melt olive oil and 1 ounce beeswax together in double boiler; stir in tea and simmer until water has evaporated. Add more beeswax if necessary. Add essential oil and about 4 drops of tincture of Benzoin (a preservative). Store in cool place in dark jar.*

Matching Type of Preparation to Application

Buying echinacea products in the United States is a matter of choosing among a very limited number of kinds of products: tinctures, liquid extracts, encapsulated powders and creams. There are good, bad and indifferent products in each category. It is beyond the scope of this booklet to make specific recommendations. The following chart is designed as a guide in choosing the proper form for a specific purpose. The reader must decide whether to prepare the product him/herself, or find a trustworthy brand name.

---

*Procedure based on material found in Nuzzi, D., *Herbal Preparations and Natural Therapies*, Morning Star Publications, Boulder, Colorado.

MATCHING ECHINACEA PREPARATIONS TO APPLICATIONS

Preparation	Application
Capsule, whole powdered plant	Tonic; increases natural, nonspecific resistance to disease; daily consumption okay. Good for allergies.
Tincture of root or dried tops, or both	Acute internal or external infections or inflammations. Intermittent use, as necessary.
Liquid extract of root or dried tops or both	Acute infections, especially systemic; intermittent use required.
Ointment/Salve/Cream/Lotion	External wounds, infections, sores, eczema, psoriasis, burns, herpes simplex, candida. Use as needed.

POLITICS: THEN AND NOW

The political history of echinacea, previously discussed, has clearly demonstrated how the American Medical Association has used non-medical means to destroy an entire school of medicine along with its methods and medicines. Today the political issues, represented by the strength of the AMA and tenor of the current FDA regulations, continue to limit the ability of proponents of natural, non-intrusive medicine and health maintenance to educate the public on alternative methods and medicines. Alternative medicine is caught in a political "catch-22." Unable to acquire government money to research medical claims for natural products, alternative practitioners are prevented from making even limited, common-sense claims for such materials.

The public must rely on books such as this, some written by non-professionals and worse, as the source of their education. Few professionals are willing to risk reputation and livelihood by writing on "unproven" practices, even when they know them to be safe and effective.

Thus modern medicine continues to rely on seriously flawed medication such as antibiotics to treat ailments that really require immunotonics, cardiotonics, digestive tonics and other mild, natural materials. Deprived of substances that simply increase the body's own ability to mend itself and keep itself healthy, modern orthodox doctors continue to administer intrusive, synthetic, powerful drugs that are totally inappropriate to the needs of the patient, and which, after brief periods of use, actually cause the body to develop immunity to their impact, thus demanding an ever growing number of intrusive drugs which eventually destroy the body's natural immune responses.

Despite the fact that echinacea is growing in popularity even among orthodox physicians who privately use it instead of drugs, but are not allowed to recommend it to their patients, the political climate in this country continues to lag behind its counterparts in many other countries. Professionals from Europe and Asia often express amazement at the naive, mean-spirited, and unenlightened nature of American medicine, where economic, educational, political and medical repression rules the day. Let us hope for a future in which these wrongs are corrected, and all people are allowed access to simple substances like echinacea that will dramatically increase the individual's ability to maintain tone and balance in the body systems, reduce the number of visits to the doctor's office and lower our overall health care costs at the same time.

REFERENCES

The Echinacea Story—A History

1. Lloyd, J.U. "Empiricism—Echinacea." *The Eclectic Medical Journal*, LVII(8), 1–7, 1897.
2. Excerpted from Lloyd, J.U. Ibid.
3. Felter, H.W., M.D. "The newer materia medica. I. Echinacea." *The Eclectic Medical Journal*, LVIII(2), 79, 1898.

4. Felter, H.W., M.D. Ibid., pp. 79–89.
5. Felter, H.W., M.D. *Echinacea*. Lloyd Bros. Pharmacists, Inc., Cincinnati, Ohio, probably somewhere between 1900 and 1905.
6. Rounseville, G.L.B., M.D. "Echinacca angustifolia radix de candolle." Read at a joint meeting of the Wood, Clark, Portage and Taylor Counties and Northwestern Wisconsin Medical Societies, Marshfield, Wisconsin, February 5, 1907.
7. Lloyd, J.U. "Vegetable drugs employed by American physicians." *The Journal of the American Pharmaceutical Association*, November 1912.
8. Fearn, J. "Echinacea." *The Eclectic Medical Journal*, LXXIV(4), 177–181, 1914.
9. von Unruh, V. "Echinacea Angustifolia and Inula Helenium in the treatment of tuberculosis." *National Eclectic Medical Association Quarterly*, September 1915.
10. *The Gleaner*, February 1928, pp. 1053–1054.
11. Waterhouse, Dr. E.R. in *The Eclectic Medical Gleaner*, reprinted in *The Eclectic Medical Journal*, November 1896.
12. Editorial in *The Eclectic Medical Journal*, November 1896.
13. Kilgour, J.C., M.D., Harrison, Ohio, in *The Eclectic Medical Journal*, November 1897.
14. Scudder, J.M. *The Essential Differences Between the Three Schools of Medicine: Allopathic, Eclectic and Homeopathic*. Published by the House of Lloyd, Cincinnati, Ohio.
15. Editorial. *Journal of the American Medical Association*, November 27, 1909, p. 1836.
16. Editorial. *Journal of the American Medical Association*, February 27, 1909, pp. 720–721.
17. Couch, J.F., and Giltner, L.T. "An experimental study of echinacea therapy." *Journal of Agricultural Research*, 20, 63–84, 1920.
18. Beal, J.H. "Summary of the physiological report of Couch and Giltner." *American Journal of Pharmacy*, 93, 229–232, 1921.
19. Niederkorn, J.S. *A Handy Reference Book*. Lloyd Bros., Cincinnati, Ohio, 1930.
20. Cutler, S.H. and Fellow, L. "Echinacea: A phytochemical study." *Bulletin of the University of Wisconsin*, Serial No. 1787, General Series No. 1571, Madison, Wisconsin, 1931.

1. Bonadeo, I., Bottazzi, G. and Lavazza, M. "Echinacin B: Polisaccaride attivo dell' echinacea." *Riv. Ital. Essenze Profumi*, 53, 281, 1971.
2. Chone, B. "Gezielte steuerung der leukozytentinetik durch echinacin." *Arzneimittel-Forschung*, 11, 611, 1965.
3. Buesing, K. H. "Inhibition of hyaluronidase by echinacin." *Arzneimittel Forschung*, 2, 467–469, 1952.
4. Koch, E. and Uebel, H. "Experimental studies concerning the local action of echinacea purpurea or tissues." *Arzneimittel Forschung*, 3, 16–19, 1953.
5. Kuhn, O. "Echinacea and phagocytosis." *Arzneimittel Forschung*, 3, 194–200, 1953.
6. Tuennerhoff, F. K., and Schwabe, H. K. "Untersuchungen am menschen und am tier ueber den einfluss von echinaceakonzentraten auf die kuenstliche bindergewebsbildung nach fibrin-implantationen." *Arzneimittel Forschung*, 6(6), 330–334, 1956.
7. Vogel, G., et al. "Evaluation of anitexudative drugs." *Arzneimittel Forschung*, 18(4), 426–429, 1968.
8. Viehmann, P. *Erfahrungsheilkunde*, 27(6), 353–358, 1978.
9. Mund-Hoym, W.D. *Aerztliche Praxis*, 31(14), 566–567, 1979.
10. Sickel, K. *Aerztliche Praxis*, 23, 201, 1971.
11. Kinkel, H. J., Plate, M., and Tuellner, U. *Med. Klinik*, 79(21), 580–583, 1984.
12. Quadripur, S. A. *Therapie der Gegenwart*, 115, 1072, 1976.
13. Wacker, A., and Hilbig, A. "Virus inhibition by echinacea purpurea." *Planta Medica*, 33, 89–102, 1978.
14. Schnurbusch, F. Z. *Laryng. Rhinol. Otol.*, 34, 520, 1955.
15. Koring, G. W., and Born, W. *Arzneimittel Forschung*, 4, 424–426, 1954.
16. Koring, G. W., and Rasp, K. *Medizinische Welt*, 45, 1504–1508, 1954.
17. Gaertner, W. *Landartz*, 39(3), 123–124, 1963.
18. Viehmann, P. *op. cit.*
19. Mund-Hoym, W. D. *op. cit.*
20. Chone, B., & Manidakis, G. *Deutscher Medizinische Wochenschrift*, 27, 1406, 1969.
21. Viehmann, P. *op. cit.*
22. Kinkel, H. J., Plate, M., and Tuellner, U. *op. cit.*
23. Foster, S. *Echinacea: Nature's Immune Enhancer*, Healing Arts Press, Rochester, Vermont, 1991.

24. Hobbs, C. *The Echinacea Handbook*, Eclectic Medical Publications, Portland, Oregon, 1989.

25. Stimpel, M., Proksh, A., Wagner, H., and Lohmann-Matthes, M.L. "Macrophage activation and induction of macrophage cytotoxicity by purified polysaccharide fractions from the plant *Echinacea purpurea.*" *Infection and Immunity*, 46(3), 845–849, 1984.

26. Wagner, H., et al. "Immunstimulierend wirkende polysaccaride (Heteroglykane) aus hoeheren plfanzen." *Arzneimittel Forschung*, 34, 659–661, 1984.

27. Kuhn, O. *Arzneimittel Forschung*, 3, 194, 1953.

28. Wagner, H., and Proksch, A. "An immunostimulating active principle from *Echinacea purpurea.*" *Zeitschrift fuer Angewandte Phyotherapie*, 2(5), 166–168, 171, 1981.

29. Wagner, H., and Proksch, A. "Isolation of polysaccharides with immunostimulating activity from *Echinacea purpurea.*" *International Conference Chem. Biotechnil. Biol. Act. Nat. Prod. (Proceedings)*, Atanasova, B., ed. 3(1), 200–202, 1981.

30, Bauer, R., and Wagner, H. *Echinacea Handbuch fuer Aerzte, Apotheker und andere Naturwissenschaftler.* Stuttgart, Germany, Wissenschaftliche Verlagsgesellschaft mbH., 1990.

31. Buesing, H. K. "Die beeinflussung des properdin-spiegels durch extrakte aus echinacea purpurea bei kannichen." *Zhurnal Immunitaetsforschung*, 115, 169–176, 1958.

32. Orinda, D., Diederich, J., and Wacker, A. "Antiviral activity of constituents of *Echinacea purpurea.*" *Arzneimittel Forschung*, 23 (8), 1119–1120, 1973.

33. Von Eilmes, H. G. *Dissertation*, Frankfurt/M., Germany, 1976.

34. Wacker, A., and Hilbig, A. "Virus inhibition by *Echinacea purpurea.*" *Planta Medica*, 33, 89–102, 1978.

35. Wagner, H., and Proksch, A. *op. cit.*

36. Coeuginiet, E., and Kuehnast, R. "Recurrent candidiasis: adjuvant immunotherapy with different formulations of echinacin." *Therapiewoche*, 36(33), 3352–3358, 1986.

37. Stoll, A., Renz, A., and Brack, A. "Antibacterial substances II. Isolation and constitution of echinacoside, a glycoside from the roots of *Echinacea angustifolia.*" *Helvetic Chimica Acta*, 33, 1877–1893, 1950.

38. Becker, V. H. "Against snakebites and influenza; use and components of *Echinacea angustifolia* and *E. purpurea.*" *Deutsche Apotheker Zeitung*, 122(45), 2020–2323, 1982.

39. Koch, E., and Uebel, H. "Experimental studies concerning the local action of *Echinacea purpurea* on tissues." *Arzneimittel Forschung*, 3, 16–19, 1953.

40. Koch, E., and Hasse, H. "A modification of the spreading test in animal assays." *Arzneimittel Forschung*, 2, 454–467, 1952.
41. Koch, E., and Uebel, H. "Experimental studies on the local influence of cortisone and echinacin upon tissue resistance against streptococcus infection." *Arzneimittel Forschung*, 4, 424–426, 1954.
42. Kleinschmidt, H. *Therapie der Gegenwart*, 104, 1258–1262, 1965.
43. Freyer, H. U. *Fortschritte der Medizin*, 52, 165–168, 1974.
44. Messner, F. K. *Die Therapiewoche*, 9, 522–523, 1951.
45. Volz, G. *Therapie der Gegenwart*, 98 (8), 1957.
46. Zimmerman, O. *Hippokrates*, 40(6), 233–235, 1969.
47. Baetgen, D. *Therapiewoche*, 34(36), 5115–5119, 1984.
48. Keller, H., Inventor. "Recovery of active agents from aqueous extracts of the species of echinacea." Chemie Gruenenthal G.M.B.H., GER. 950,674, Oct. 11, 1956.
49. Bonadeio, I., Bottazi, G., and Lavazza, M. "Echinacina B: polisaccaride attivo dell echinacea." *Rev. Ital. Essenze Profumi*, 53, 281, 1971.
50. Bonadeo, I., and Lavazza, M. "Echinacina B: suo azione sui fibroblasti." *Riv. Ital. Essenze Profumi*, 54, 195, 1972.
51. Tragini, E., Tubaro, A., Melis, S., and Galli, L. "Evidence from two classic irritation tests for an anti-inflammatory action of a natural extract, echinacina B." *Food and Chemical Toxicology*, 23(2), 317–319, 1985.
52. Seidel, K. & Knobloch, H. "Proof and comparison of the anti-phlogistic effect of antirheumatic drugs." *Zhurnal der Rheumaforschung*, 16, 231–238, 1957.
53. Vogel, G., et. al. "Evaluation of antiexudative drugs." *Arzneimittel Forschung*, 18(4), 426–429, 1968.
54. Tubaro, A., Tragni, E., Del Negro, P., et al. "Anti-inflammatory activity of a polysaccharide fraction of *Echinacea angustifolia*." *J. Pharm. Pharmacol.*, 39, 567–569, 1986.
55. Voaden, D. J., and Jacobson, M. "Tumor-inhibitors III. Identification and synthesis of an oncolytic hydrocarbon from American coneflower roots." *Journal of Medicinal Chemistry*, 15(6), 619–623, 1972.
56. Fong, B., et al. *Lloydia*, 35, 38, 1972.
57. Lasche, H. G. *Die Med. Welt*, 34, 1463, 1983.